NATURAL WAYS TO FERTILITY ENHANCEMENT WITH HERBS

Herbal Harmony, Unveiling The Secrets To Assisted Reproductive Technology Through Natural Remedies

DR. JEREMY ALLEY

Disclaimer:

The information provided in this book, is intended for general informational purposes only and should not be considered as professional advice.

The author has made every effort to ensure the accuracy of the information presented. However, readers are advised to consult with a qualified healthcare professional before attempting any herbal remedies or making significant changes to their wellness routine. Individual health conditions vary, and what may be suitable for one person may not be appropriate for another.

It is important to note that the author is not in any endorsement deal, partnership, or affiliation with any organization, brand, or company mentioned in this book. Any references to specific products or services are based on the author's personal experience or general knowledge and do not imply an endorsement or promotion of those products or services.

Contents

Recognition Of Fertility

The capacity to conceive and bring a baby to term is known as fertility, and it is a complicated component of reproductive health. Fertility can be difficult for both men and women to achieve or maintain, and this can be influenced by several factors, including age, lifestyle, and general health. For those looking for natural solutions to increase their reproductive capacity, it is essential to comprehend the complexities of fertility.

Fundamentals of the Reproductive Systems of Men and Women

Understanding the basic functioning of the male and female reproductive systems is necessary to understand fertility enhancement. Fertility in women is mostly dependent on the menstrual cycle, ovulation, and uterine health. For effective reproduction, however, men need the generation of healthy sperm. Understanding these systems' complexities lays the groundwork for resolving fertility issues and putting natural solutions into practice.

Variables Impacting Fertility

Fertility can be affected by a wide range of variables, from underlying medical issues to lifestyle decisions. Given that both men's and women's fertility tends to decrease with age, age is a crucial variable. Infertility issues can also be caused by nutritional deficiencies, stress, and hormonal abnormalities. Reproductive health may suffer from exposure to chemicals and other environmental causes. Comprehending these elements is essential for spotting any roadblocks and creating all-encompassing strategies to improve fertility organically.

Herbs to Boost Female Fertility

For ages, people from diverse cultures have used herbs to promote the reproductive health of women. Certain herbs are thought to help women become more fertile overall, encourage ovulation, and manage their menstrual cycles. Maca root (Lepidium meyenii), red clover (Trifolium pratense), and chasteberry (Vitex agnus-castus) are a few examples. These herbs are believed to help uterine health, regulate hormones, and treat underlying problems that could prevent conception.

Herbs to Boost Male Fertility

Herbal treatments to improve fertility can also be beneficial for men. It is believed that several herbs can increase sperm motility, increase sperm production, and improve male reproductive health in general. Herbs that are frequently used to increase male fertility include ashwagandha (Withania somnifera), maca root, and Tribulus terrestris. It is thought that these herbs enhance sperm quality, lower oxidative stress, and strengthen the endocrine system, all of which promote fertility.

Nutrition-Based Methods to Increase Fertility

The foundation of reproductive health is appropriate nutrition. A balanced diet full of vital nutrients promotes men's and women's general health and has a good impact on fertility.

Antioxidants, omega-3 fatty acids, zinc, and folate are important nutrients. Fertility-promoting foods including leafy greens, nuts, seeds, and fatty fish can be incorporated into a diet to improve reproductive health and correct any nutritional deficiencies that may be impeding fertility.

Lifestyle Adjustments to Boost Fertility

Fertility is greatly influenced by lifestyle choices, and adopting healthy lifestyle modifications can naturally increase fertility.

Crucial components include stress management, frequent physical activity, and maintaining a healthy weight. Reproductive health can be adversely affected by tobacco use, excessive alcohol use, and the use of illegal substances.

Therefore, it is imperative to avoid them. A favorable environment for maximum fertility can be created by including stress-relieving activities, enough sleep, and mindfulness techniques in everyday life.

Conventional Methods and Holistic Approaches

Holistic methods of enhancing fertility combine traditional techniques, nutrition, and lifestyle choices.

One traditional Chinese medicine method that is thought to control energy flow and enhance reproductive health is acupuncture.

The benefits of yoga and meditation in lowering stress are also widely accepted. Completing a fertility enhancement plan with these holistic activities can offer a well-rounded approach to managing the mental and physical components of reproductive health.

CHAPTER ONE

OVERVIEW OF HERBAL MEDICINE

For millennia, people have turned to herbal medicine as a natural way to address specific health issues and promote general health.

Herbs have become more well-known in the field of reproductive health because of their ability to increase fertility.

For individuals looking for natural solutions to increase fertility, it's imperative to comprehend the fundamentals of herbal medicine.

Herbs are plant-based medications that have a variety of chemicals that may have therapeutic benefits.

These substances can affect hormone balance, strengthen the uterus, and improve reproductive function in general.

Selecting The Best Herbs To Increase Fertility

The distinct health requirements and fertility issues of each individual must be carefully considered while choosing the right herbs for enhancing fertility.

Herbs have long been used to treat a variety of reproductive health issues, including regulating menstrual cycles, enhancing the quality of eggs, and maintaining a healthy uterine environment. Herbs like Vitex (Chaste Tree), Maca root, Red Clover, and Dong Quai are frequently suggested for fertility.

To make sure that herbs are compatible with specific medical problems and drugs, it is essential to speak with a certified herbalist or healthcare expert before introducing any herbs into a reproductive routine.

Menstrual Cycle Regulation With Herbs

Menstrual cycle irregularities may make it more difficult to conceive. It has been discovered that several herbs can control menstrual cycles, hence fostering hormonal equilibrium.

Vitex, sometimes referred to as the Chaste Tree, is frequently advised for this use. By affecting the pituitary gland, which is essential for controlling hormones, it might aid with menstrual cycle regulation.

Herbs like wild yam and black cohosh may also be taken into consideration for their ability to promote menstrual regularity.

Enhancing The Quality Of Eggs Via Herbal Supplements

Fertility is greatly influenced by the quality of the eggs, particularly in women who are trying to become pregnant. Traditional medicine has employed herbal supplements, such as maca root, to improve reproductive health, particularly the quality of eggs.

Nutrient- and adaptogenic-rich maca root may help regulate hormones and promote healthy reproduction in general. A balanced diet that includes maca root may help to improve egg quality, which may raise the likelihood of a successful conception.

Red Clover: Boosting Uterine Health

A healthy uterus is essential to a fruitful pregnancy. Herb red clover is well-known for its ability to promote uterine health. It contains substances like isoflavones that may function similarly to estrogen and support a healthy uterine environment. Red clover is a common ingredient in herbal remedies meant to promote fertility by fostering the best conditions possible for the implantation and growth of embryos.

Dong Quai and Hormone Balancing

Fertility depends on hormonal balance, which is why traditional Chinese medicine frequently uses the herb dong quai to treat hormonal imbalances. The adaptogenic qualities of this plant are thought to help control estrogen levels and promote hormonal balance in general. Dong Quai should, however, be used carefully and under a doctor's supervision as overindulgence may have negative consequences.

Using Herbs In Everyday Living

Integrating the right herbs into daily life is crucial for enhancing fertility after they have been found. There are several ways to accomplish this, such as using tinctures, supplements, or herbal teas. Fertility-enhancing herb teas might be a tasty and practical way to incorporate these plants into your everyday routine.

Concentrated liquid extracts called tinctures provide a practical solution for accurate dosage.

For safety and efficacy, it is essential to adhere to suggested dosages and guidelines.

Herbs provide a safe, natural way to increase fertility, but it's important to use them carefully and under a doctor's supervision.

Herbs can have different effects on different people, and some may interfere with prescription drugs or pre-existing medical issues.

The combination of conventional wisdom and contemporary medical understanding can offer a thorough approach to improving fertility, guaranteeing a well-rounded and knowledgeable plan for individuals looking for natural options while trying to conceive.

CHAPTER TWO

HERBS FOR THE FERTILITY OF WOMEN

For millennia, people have used herbs to treat a variety of health issues, including infertility. Certain herbs are thought to provide natural support for improving women's fertility. These herbs can be divided into groups according to how they specifically affect certain facets of reproductive health.

Using Herbs To Control Menstrual Cycles

Menstrual cycle regulation is essential for maximizing fertility. Women who experience irregular menstrual cycles may find it difficult to conceive since it may throw off the timing of ovulation.

Numerous herbs are well-known for their ability to naturally control menstrual periods. One common herb in this category is vitex, sometimes referred to as chasteberry. It is thought to increase luteinizing hormone (LH) production, which is important for controlling the menstrual cycle. Furthermore, a traditional Chinese herb called dong quai is frequently used to treat disorders like amenorrhea and promote regular menstruation.

Herbal Remedies For Ovulation

Fertility relies heavily on ovulation because it is during this stage that the egg leaves the ovary and becomes ready for fertilization. It's well known that several herbs can help and promote ovulation. The Peruvian native maca root is said to help regulate hormones and encourage regular ovulation.

Another herb that may promote the synthesis of hormones like luteinizing hormone (LH), which is necessary for ovulation, is Tribulus terrestris, which is frequently used in traditional medicine.

Herbs To Promote Better Fetal Health

A successful conception and a healthy pregnancy depend on a healthy uterus. Fertilized eggs can be implanted more easily in an environment that is optimally created by herbs that promote uterine health. Vitamin and mineral-rich raspberry leaf is a well-known plant for toning the uterine muscles and enhancing general uterine health. Because red clover contains phytoestrogen, it's thought to help maintain a healthy uterine lining. Furthermore, the nutrient-rich nettle leaf may support a healthy and functional uterus.

While these herbs are frequently used in traditional medicine, there is conflicting scientific evidence about their effectiveness in enhancing fertility. People should speak with a healthcare provider before adding herbal therapies to a reproductive regimen, particularly if there are any underlying medical disorders or concerns.

Herbs can be very helpful allies when trying to increase fertility organically.

These herbs have been used by many to supplement traditional reproductive treatments, whether they are supporting normal menstruation, encouraging ovulation, or fostering uterine health. The safety and efficacy of herbal remedies depend on tailored advice from medical professionals, just like any other health-related undertaking.

CHAPTER THREE

HERBS FOR THE FERTILITY OF MEN

Many individuals and couples who want to start a family worry about their fertility. Even though there are medical options, some people use natural solutions to increase their fertility.

Herbs have been used traditionally for their possible advantages; this is one area of investigation. Certain herbs are thought to help with sperm quality, count, and general reproductive health when it comes to men's fertility.

Herbs To Boost Sperm Count And Quality

Tribulus Terrestris: This herb has been used for a very long time in traditional medicine, and it is believed to increase male fertility by increasing the motility and count of sperm.

Moreover, Tribulus terrestris may support hormonal homeostasis by raising testosterone levels.

Maca Root: Known for its adaptogenic qualities, maca root is said to promote the health of male reproduction.

It might improve the motility, quantity, and general quality of sperm. Maca is also believed to assist in balancing hormones and reducing stress, both of which may have an indirect effect on fertility.

Ashwagandha: This adaptogenic herb has been linked to better sperm parameters. Research indicates that it might raise testosterone levels, sperm count, and motility. Moreover, ashwagandha has a reputation for lowering stress, which may enhance fertility by lessening the damaging effects of stress.

Ginseng: Traditionally, ginseng—specifically, Panax ginseng—has been used to enhance male reproduction. It might have a favorable effect on the motility and morphology of sperm. Additionally known for its adaptogenic properties, ginseng may help support healthy reproduction in general.

Saw Palmetto: Saw palmetto is frequently used to treat prostate issues, but it may also increase male fertility. It is thought to promote healthy prostate function, which benefits reproductive health in general. Some studies suggest that saw palmetto may improve sperm parameters, but additional research is required.

Herbs To Improve The Health Of Male Reproduction

Mucuna Pruriens: Known by other names as velvet bean, this herb has an L-DOPA precursor that leads to dopamine. Mucuna pruriens may increase testosterone levels and sperm quality, which may support male fertility.

Additionally, sperm may be shielded from oxidative damage by its antioxidant qualities.

Nettle Root: Nettle root has long been utilized to treat a range of male health issues, including reproductive system-related issues. It is believed to regulate hormones and promote prostate health, which may improve male reproductive health in general.

Ginkgo Biloba: Well-known for enhancing cognitive function, ginkgo biloba may help increase male fertility. It is thought to increase blood flow, which might boost the function of the reproductive organs. Furthermore, the antioxidant qualities of ginkgo biloba might shield sperm from oxidative damage.

Horny Goat Weed: This herb has been used for many years to promote male reproductive health as well as other health issues in traditional Chinese medicine. It might enhance libido and erectile function, which might aid in fertility.

Red Clover: Isoflavones, which are found in red clover, are thought to have properties similar to those of estrogen. Some studies suggest that red clover may help male fertility by promoting hormonal balance; however, additional research is needed to confirm these claims.

Herbs are sometimes thought of as a natural way to increase fertility, but it's important to use caution when using them.

Before adding herbs to a reproductive program, it is best to speak with a healthcare provider, especially if the person is taking medication or has pre-existing medical conditions.

In addition, maintaining a nutritious diet, getting regular exercise, and managing stress are important lifestyle choices that support overall reproductive well-being.

CHAPTER FOUR

CHANGES IN LIFESTYLE FOR FERTILITY

Starting a quest to improve fertility frequently necessitates substantial lifestyle adjustments. These adjustments cover a wide range of day-to-day activities, such as stress reduction, exercise, and diet. People can foster an atmosphere that promotes reproductive health and raises the chance of conception by taking a holistic approach.

Tips For Diet And Nutrition

An essential component of naturally boosting fertility is keeping a nutrient-rich, well-balanced diet. Essential minerals and vitamins are critical to reproductive health.

 Eating a diet high in antioxidant-rich foods, like fruits and vegetables, can help prevent oxidative stress and support a fertile environment. Men and women alike must also make sure they are getting enough folate, iron, and other important nutrients.

The Effects Of Exercise On Fertility

Frequent exercise has major positive effects on fertility in addition to being good for general health. Moderate exercise helps maintain a healthy body weight, enhance blood circulation, and balance hormones—all of which have a good impact on reproductive health.

But it's important to find a balance because too much exercise might negatively impact fertility. Moderation is key when it comes to physical activity.

Techniques For Stress Management

Stress affects both men and women and can be a significant barrier to conception. Establishing a suitable atmosphere for conception requires the implementation of appropriate stress management measures.

Stress reduction techniques include yoga, deep breathing exercises, and meditation. Furthermore, making time for leisure and participation in happy and fulfilling pursuits can enhance general well-being and have a favorable impact on reproductive health.

Developing a balanced lifestyle that includes these three pillars—exercise, stress reduction, and nutrition—can dramatically increase fertility naturally.

It's critical to understand that it could take some time for these adjustments to take effect and that maintaining consistency is essential to enjoying the full benefits of a fertility-focused lifestyle.

CHAPTER FIVE

HERBAL CURES AND MANUFACTURERS

Many resort to natural therapies, especially herbs, to promote reproductive health in their quest for increased fertility. These herbs are said to have the ability to balance hormones, enhance the menstrual cycle, and treat underlying fertility-related conditions. Including herbal treatments in one's regimen is sometimes regarded as a comprehensive strategy for improving fertility.

Herbal Fertility Teas

For generations, herbal teas have been utilized as a calming and healing elixir, and some are even thought to increase fertility.

For example, red clover tea is believed to support hormonal balance, and nettle tea is a great source of iron and vitamin K.

Another well-liked option is raspberry leaf tea, which is well-known for its ability to enhance general reproductive health and tone the uterine muscles. These herbal teas are a reassuring and maybe helpful complement to the fertility journey, and they are simple to incorporate into a daily routine.

Herbal Tinctures And Infusions

Herbal tinctures and infusions provide additional ways to utilize the fertility-boosting properties of herbs besides drinks.

The Peruvian herb maca root is used frequently in fertility infusions because of its adaptogenic qualities, which are thought to aid in hormone balance.

Vitex, sometimes referred to as chasteberry, is another herb that is frequently made into a tincture and is believed to help women's hormonal balance.

These tinctures and infusions can be customized to meet specific needs, providing a flexible way to incorporate herbal treatments into a program centered around fertility.

Recipes For Fertility-Boosting Smoothies

Smoothies that are high in nutrients offer a tasty and practical method to include fertility-enhancing herbs in the diet. In addition to being high in vitamins and minerals, green smoothies made with components like kale and spinach can also incorporate herbs like spirulina or maca to enhance fertility. In addition to herbs like red clover or dong quai, fruits like berries—which are noted for their antioxidant qualities—may also be included in a fertility smoothie.

For individuals seeking to improve fertility through food, these smoothie recipes provide a satisfying and healthy choice.

Before adding herbs to a fertility regimen, like with any natural medicine, it is important to speak with a healthcare provider, particularly if there are any underlying medical disorders or concerns.

Additionally, the use of herbal treatments in supporting overall reproductive wellness is complemented by maintaining a healthy lifestyle that includes frequent exercise, a balanced diet, and stress management.

Herbs can be a useful ally in the quest for increased fertility, but individual reactions might differ, thus for best effects, a comprehensive approach to reproductive health is advised.

CHAPTER SIX

AVOIDANCE AND RECOMMENDATIONS

It is important to think about any possible dangers and contraindications before adding herbs to a fertility-enhancing program.

Although most people think herbs are safe, certain people may have negative interactions or effects.

Speaking With A Medical Professional

It is strongly advised that you speak with a healthcare provider before beginning any natural fertility treatment.

A medical professional can evaluate a patient's unique medical history, current prescriptions, and other risk factors to provide tailored advice regarding the suitability and safety of herbal supplements.

The combination of herbs and pharmaceuticals may alter their effectiveness or result in unfavorable side effects.

Notifying medical professionals about the use of any herbs, vitamins, or prescription drugs is crucial. By being proactive, any interactions that can hurt reproductive health are avoided.

An all-natural and comprehensive approach to fertility enhancement may involve the use of herbs. Herbal medicines should be used cautiously, nevertheless, taking into account specific medical problems and any drug combinations.

A targeted, educated approach that involves consultation with medical professionals guarantees a secure and efficient path to better fertility.

CHAPTER SEVEN

ACHIEVEMENT AND WHOLE HEALTH

A complicated element of human health, fertility is influenced by several physiological, psychological, and environmental variables.

It is frequently necessary to take a holistic approach to achieving optimal fertility, taking into account both mental and physical health.

Growing interest has been seen in the use of natural medicines, especially herbs, to improve fertility in recent years. These herbs are thought to complement holistic methods in a complementary way, addressing the mind-body link as well as the physical components of fertility.

Combining Herbs And Holistic Methods

Holistic approaches to fertility place a strong emphasis on the connections between several facets of health, such as lifestyle, nutrition, and mental health. Including herbs in these methods can offer a comprehensive plan for improving fertility.

Herbs like Vitex agnus-castus, or chasteberry, are thought to help maintain hormonal balance, for example. This herb has been used traditionally to treat irregular periods and to control menstrual cycles.

Maca root is another herb that is frequently included in holistic reproductive methods. Maca is thought to enhance libido and affect hormonal balance. It is frequently used to enhance sperm and egg quality as well as general reproductive health. Maca's adaptogenic qualities are believed to aid the body in adjusting to stress, which may be a factor in infertility problems.

Herbal blends, as opposed to single herbs, are becoming more and more well-liked for supporting fertility. Several plants are often combined in these mixtures for complimentary benefits. For instance, a combination might contain fertility-specific herbs like Tribulus terrestris with adaptogenic herbs like Rhodiola rosea and ashwagandha. These combos try to address stress management and hormone balance, among other elements of fertility.

The Mind-Body Link In Fertility

Fertility is greatly impacted by the mind-body relationship since emotional stability and stress levels can affect reproductive health. Herbal medicine can be used in conjunction with holistic therapies such as yoga, mindfulness, and meditation. Herbs with adaptogenic qualities, including holy basil (tulsi), are frequently suggested to assist the body in managing stress.

It is thought that these herbs can regulate the stress response, which could lead to better reproductive outcomes.

In addition, herbal teas with calming properties like lemon balm and chamomile can help promote a healthy mind-body connection. In addition to being calming, these teas allow people a chance to include mindful rituals in their everyday lives.

Combining herbal remedies with holistic methods provides a complete plan for improving fertility. By attending to the mental and physical facets of reproductive health, people can establish an atmosphere that is conducive to conception.

But, it's crucial to approach these treatments holistically, understanding that fertility is impacted by a multitude of circumstances that go beyond the usage of herbs.

Before adding herbs to your fertility routine, always get medical advice, especially if you are taking medication or have underlying medical conditions.

CHAPTER EIGHT

GETTING READY FOR MATERNITY

Pregnancy planning for couples intending to have children requires a comprehensive strategy that takes into account many facets of lifestyle and health. Understanding fertility and implementing actions that improve reproductive health are essential components of this process. Utilizing natural remedies, such as herbs, can be very beneficial for promoting fertility.

Establishing A Fertility-Friendly Ambience

Enhancing one's physical and mental health is essential to establishing a fertility-friendly atmosphere. To maintain general health and fertility, a diet rich in important vitamins and minerals must be balanced and nutritious. In addition, keeping a healthy weight, controlling stress, and minimizing exposure to environmental pollutants are all essential components in fostering a fertile environment. Herbs having adaptogenic qualities, such as holy basil and ashwagandha, can help with stress management and hormone balance.

Knowing About Fertility Charts And Ovulation

To maximize the odds of conception, one must have a thorough understanding of the menstrual cycle, especially ovulation. To improve reproductive health, herbal therapies can be incorporated into the fertility charting process.

Herbs with the reputation of regulating menstrual periods and supporting general hormonal balance include a chaste tree (Vitex agnus-castus). To determine viable periods and optimal timing for sexual activity, couples might utilize herbal supplements in conjunction with fertility charting techniques, such as monitoring changes in cervical mucus and basal body temperature.

Herbs To Increase Fertility

Numerous herbs are well known for their ability to naturally increase fertility. Because of its adaptogenic qualities, maca root is said to enhance reproductive health and maintain hormonal balance. Another herb, Tribulus terrestris, has also been traditionally used to treat male and female infertility. Chinese herb dong quai is frequently suggested because of its ability to control menstrual cycles and enhance blood flow to the reproductive organs.

Fertility Support Through Nutrition

Fertility is greatly influenced by nutrition, and several herbs can be used to enhance a well-balanced diet. For example, red clover is high in minerals like magnesium and calcium, which encourage healthy reproduction in general. Iron and vitamin K are two of the many minerals found in nettle leaf, a nutrient-dense herb that may support a healthy reproductive system.

Herbal Infusions And Teas For Fertility

A tasty and convenient method to add fertility-boosting herbs to every day routines is through herbal teas and infusions.

One popular option is red raspberry leaf tea, which is well-known for its ability to tone the uterus.

Other herbs, like chamomile and peppermint, can be mixed to create a calming mixture that promotes both relaxation and general reproductive health.

Exercise Caution And Consult

Even while herbs can be effective allies in increasing fertility, it's important to use caution and see a specialist, particularly if there are any underlying health issues.

Speaking with a medical professional or licensed herbalist can assist in creating a customized plan that takes into account each person's unique health requirements and guarantees the safe use of herbs during the conception process.

FINAL VERDICT

Improving fertility organically calls for a multidimensional strategy that takes into account many facets of mental, emotional, and physical health.

In addition to diet, lifestyle modifications, and mind-body techniques, herbs can help maintain reproductive health.

But it's important to approach natural fertility enhancement with knowledge, and when necessary, seek expert advice.

Recap Of Important Ideas

Hormonal balance, general health, and lifestyle decisions all affect fertility.

Herbs including vitex, red clover, and maca root are said to increase fertility in women.

Herbs including Tribulus terrestris, ashwagandha, and saw palmetto may have a favorable effect on male fertility.

Adequate nutrition, including meals high in antioxidants, folic acid, and omega-3 fatty acids, promotes fertility.

A healthy weight, regular exercise, and stress reduction are all important lifestyle modifications that affect fertility.

Mind-body techniques like yoga and meditation can support healthy reproduction and help lower stress levels.

Motivation For The Upcoming Fertility Journey

Starting a fertility journey can be emotionally taxing, but people and couples can walk this route with resilience and optimism if they adopt a supportive mentality and a holistic approach. Seek advice from medical specialists, make thoughtful decisions, and keep in mind that every person's path is different. Having patience and adopting an optimistic mindset is crucial when pursuing your infertility objectives.

www.ingramcontent.com/pod-product-compliance
Lightning Source LLC
Chambersburg PA
CBHW050705250726
48662CB00002B/848